W9-AAF-565

A COLOUR ATLAS OF
DERMATOLOGY

Copyright © G M Levene & C D Calnan, 1974
Published by Wolfe Medical Publications Ltd, 1984
Printed by Grafos S.A. Arte sobre Papel,
Barcelona, Spain
17th impression 1993
ISBN 0 7234 0174 8 Cased edition
ISBN 0 7234 0863 7 Limp edition

General Editor, Wolfe Medical Books
G Barry Carruthers M D (Lond)

This book is one of the titles in the series of
Wolfe Medical Atlases, a series which brings
together probably the world's largest
systematic published collection of diagnostic
colour photographs.

For a full list of Atlases in the series, plus
forthcoming titles and details of our surgical,
dental and veterinary Atlases, please write to
Wolfe Medical Publications Ltd, Brook House.
2–16 Torrington Place, London WC1E 7LT.

All rights reserved. The contents of this book, both
photographic and textual, may not be reproduced in any
form, by print, photoprint, phototransparency, microfilm,
microfiche, or any other means, nor may it be included
in any computer retrieval system, without written
permission from the publisher.

A colour atlas
of
Dermatology

G. M. LEVENE
MB, MRCP
*Consultant Dermatologist, St John's Hospital for
Diseases of the Skin, London
Consultant Dermatologist, Middlesex Hospital, London*

&
C. D. CALNAN
MA, MB, B Chir, FRCP
*Consultant Dermatologist, St John's Hospital for
Diseases of the Skin
and The Royal Free Hospital, London*

Part 1

Wolfe Medical Publications Ltd

ACKNOWLEDGEMENTS

We wish to thank Dr R H Meara, Dean of The Institute of Dermatology and the Consultant Staff of St John's Hospital for Diseases of the Skin, London, for access to their collection of photographs. It is also a pleasure to acknowledge the help given by Mr R R Phillips, Director of the Department of Medical Illustration of the Institute, and his Staff. We are indebted to Dr H J Wallace and Dr G C Wells of St Thomas's Hospital for constant encouragement during the earliest stages of this work. For providing one or more individual photographs we are most grateful to Dr E Abell, Dr Yvonne Clayton, Dr C A Ramsay and Dr I Sarkany.

Figure **95** is from 'A Colour Atlas of Oro-Facial Diseases' by Mr L W Kay and Mr R Haskell. Figures **128**, **147** and **178** are from 'A Colour Atlas of Venereology' by Dr Anthony Wisdom.

Messrs Faber and Faber have kindly allowed us to reproduce the skin diagram which appears on page 10 in this volume. It previously appeared in 'A General Textbook of Nursing', 18th edition, by Evelyn Pearce.

To S.L. and H.L.

CONTENTS

PREFACE

Clinical dermatology is a subject in which entities tend to be well-marked and diagnosable with some precision by skilled inspection. This atlas has been prepared to help medical students, practitioners and those starting training in dermatology to become acquainted with the distinctive features of skin diseases. Most common disorders are illustrated and also several rare ones which are important with regard to associated systemic disease or to differential diagnosis. Teachers may find it useful to demonstrate features of lesions to students in their clinics.

The emphasis throughout is on diagnosis and differential diagnosis and, to facilitate this, cross-references are provided in the captions, in the introductions to sections, and in the index.

Eighty-five per cent of the photographs in this atlas were taken by the first author using a Kodak Retina Reflex III camera and Kodachrome film. The light source was a single Metz '180' flash unit. The selection of photographs necessarily reflects experience of dermatological practice in London but we believe that the range of disorders included will be helpful to practitioners in whichever community they are working.

INTRODUCTION

Modern techniques in histopathology, mycology, biochemistry, immunology and photobiology are constantly improving the accuracy of diagnosis and are expanding our understanding of the basic mechanisms of cutaneous disease. Their importance cannot be overemphasized, however at the present time it remains true that the single most useful procedure which will influence the management of patients is the visual inspection of their lesions.

It is necessary for the student to become reasonably fluent in the terms used specifically to describe skin lesions. The commonest terms are defined on pages 10–15 and some of them are illustrated by line drawings. The diagram of the vertical section of skin on page 10 shows the structural features which are referred to throughout the book. The position of pigment cells (not shown in the diagram) is described briefly on page 186.

Dermatology is particularly rich in synonyms in the nomenclature of diseases. It is best to regard many disease designations simply as code names employed to convey the concept of a pathological entity. The choice of titles used here reflects current usage in the United Kingdom. Where a title seems especially liable to mislead inverted commas are used (e.g. 'seborrhoeic' dermatitis, 'toxic' erythema).

Accurate history taking must not be neglected and should include details of the duration of the eruption, its site and mode of onset, its fluctuations with and without treatment, any skin trouble in the past, whether other members of the family or cohabitants are affected, and the presence or absence of itching and pain. Further questions will suggest themselves as the patient is examined.

If mistakes or omissions are to be avoided it will often be necessary to examine the whole of the skin surface (and mouth) in a good light, preferably daylight. The findings should be recorded in terms of (*a*) the morphology of individual lesions, (*b*) the distribution of lesions and (*c*) the arrangement or grouping of lesions. From this information diagnostic possibilities can be considered in order of probability and the need for special investigations assessed.

COMMON TERMS IN DERMATOLOGY

Dermatology, like any other speciality, has its own group of descriptive technical terms. Fortunately these are few and easily remembered.

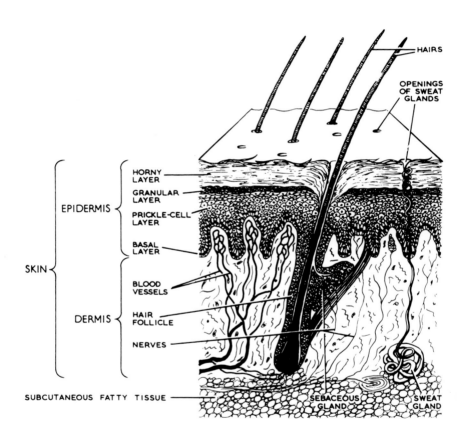

diagram of skin structure

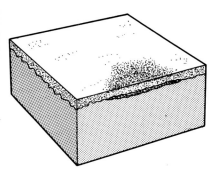

Macule A flat spot or patch of a different colour from the surrounding skin, e.g. freckles.

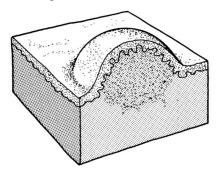

Papule A raised spot on the surface of the skin, e.g. lichen planus.

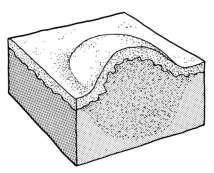

Nodule Usually indicates a lump deeply set in the skin, e.g. calcinosis.

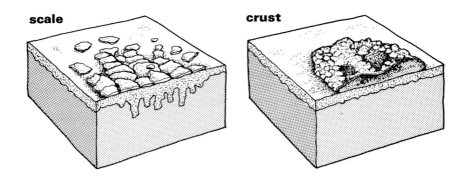

scale   **crust**

Scale A flake of flat horny cells loosened from the horny layer (stratum corneum), e.g. psoriasis.

Crust Usually refers to dried serum (serous crust), but sometimes the term is applied to a thick mass of horny cells (keratin crust) or to a mixture of both.

Pustule A skin bleb filled with pus.

Cyst A deeply situated fluid-filled cavity.

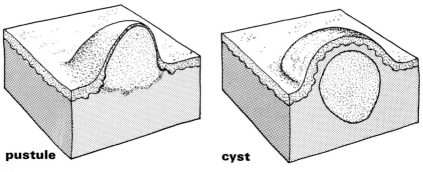

pustule   **cyst**

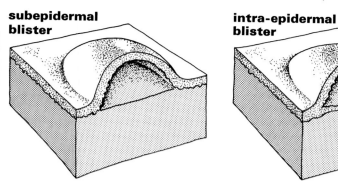

subepidermal blister

intra-epidermal blister

Blister A skin bleb filled with clear fluid. It may be :

   subepidermal, e.g. pemphigoid and dermatitis herpetiformis.

   intra-epidermal, e.g. pemphigus, eczema.

   subcorneal, e.g. impetigo.

Fissure A crack or split in the epidermis.

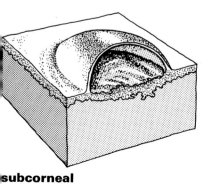

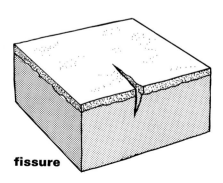

fissure

subcorneal blister

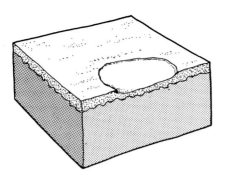

Erosion An area of partial loss of epithelium of skin or mucous membrane.

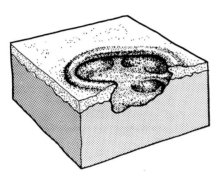

Ulcer An area of total loss of epithelium of skin or mucous membrane.

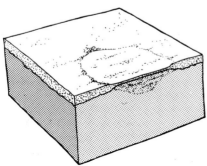

Atrophy Loss of thickness or substance of the epidermis, dermis or other tissue.

14

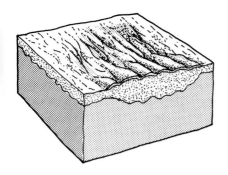

Lichenification Thickening of both the prickle-cell layer and horny layer of the epidermis with underlying inflammation giving the skin a mauvish 'morocco leather' appearance with exaggeration of normal' skin lines seen in relief, e.g. lichen simplex.

Not illustrated

Vesicle A small blister, e.g. herpes simplex, eczema.

Excoriation A scratch mark which has scored the epidermis.

Plaque A raised uniform thickening of a portion of the skin with a well-defined edge and a flat or rough surface, e.g. psoriasis.

Erythema *adj.* redness ; *noun*, an eruption with dilatation of dermal blood vessels and oedema, e.g. 'toxic' erythema.

PSORIASIS

Psoriasis is a disorder in which there is loss of control of normal epidermal cell turnover. Increased mitosis of epidermal cells results in thickening of the epidermis and the production of imperfect keratin scales. Associated with the epidermal changes are dermal vasodilatation, oedema and infiltration with polymorphonuclear leucocytes. It is not known what causes the localised disturbance of epidermal control.

1 *Psoriasis, elbows* Lesions are sharply circumscribed bright red plaques covered with coarse silvery scales. The elbows and knees are commonly involved and lesions are usually symmetrically distributed.

The cause of psoriasis is unknown. A family history of the condition is obtained in about a third of cases. Most cases begin in the second and third decade of life. It is rare below the age of five. Its course is unpredictable and lesions are usually present to a greater or lesser extent throughout life.

2 *Psoriasis* Typical small plaques showing exfoliation of silvery scales after gentle scraping with a spatula or fingernail. This is a helpful diagnostic procedure.

3 *Psoriasis, elbows* Partial treatment with ointment has cleared the scales, leaving erythematous plaques.

1

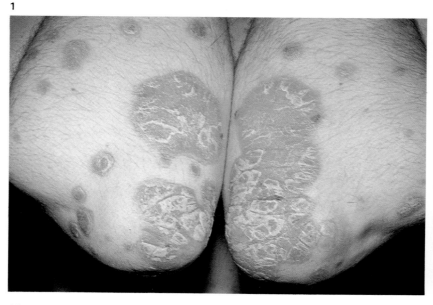

2

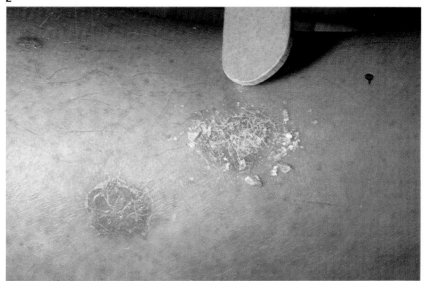

3

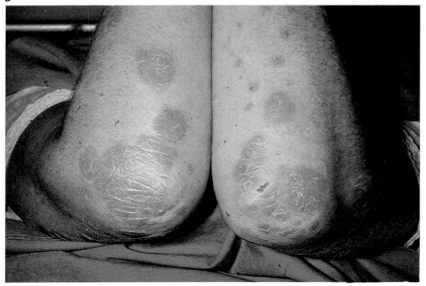

4 *Psoriasis, knees* A thick layer of keratin is obscuring underlying erythema.

5 *Psoriasis, lumbar* An extensive chronic plaque of thickened psoriasis is often found in this area.

6 *Psoriasis, Köbner phenomenon* The term 'Köbner phenomenon' means the development of a skin disease at the site of minor trauma when it is already active on other parts of the skin. This example was caused by a tight brassière and the line of psoriasis under the shoulder strap is clearly seen. Other skin diseases which are often reproduced at sites of trauma are viral warts (**142**), molluscum contagiosum (**148**) and lichen planus (**188**).

4

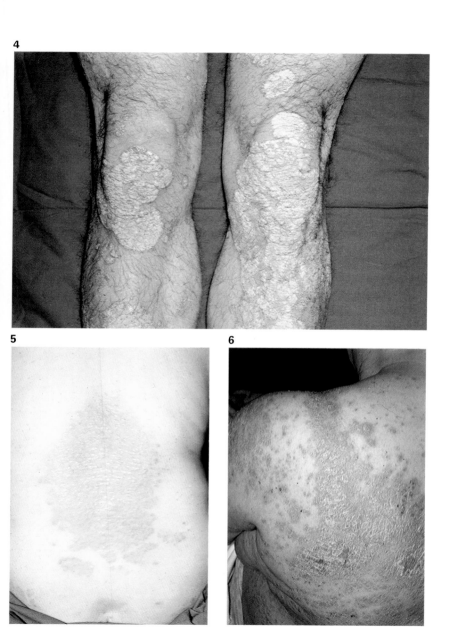

5

6

7 *Psoriasis, trunk, annular* Often plaques will heal centrally and continue to spread peripherally giving an annular configuration. Many skin diseases typically or exceptionally produce annular or arcuate lesions (see Index, 'Annular and arcuate lesions') so that this configuration is of only limited help in diagnosis.

8 *Psoriasis, flexural, perineum* Perineal, submammary and axillary psoriasis is pink, moist and glazed with minimal or absent scaling. In these situations it can be confused with candidal infection, fungal infection and other types of intertrigo. Helpful points in diagnosis are the sharply circumscribed margins of the erythema and the presence of typical psoriatic lesions elsewhere.

7

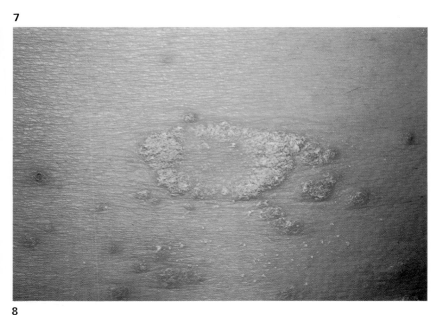

8

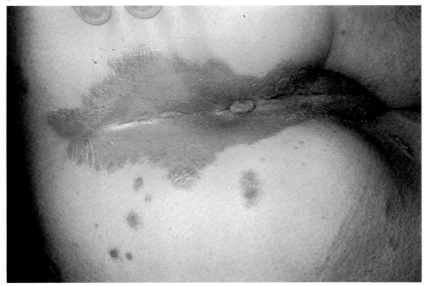

9 *Psoriasis, scalp and hair margin* The scalp is commonly affected and the presence of coarse white or yellowish-white scales in palpable plaques gives the diagnosis. There is often a tendency, as here, for the plaques to spread out beyond the hair margin. The presence of normal scalp skin between plaques distinguishes psoriasis from dandruff (pityriasis capitis) and seborrhoeic dermatitis. Visible loss of hair in psoriatic scalp plaques is uncommon.

10 *Psoriasis, nails* The fingernails show coarse 'thimble' pitting which is pathognomonic. All three nails show areas with regular pits, some of them in longitudinal formation. Nail dystrophy may be the only evidence of psoriasis.

9

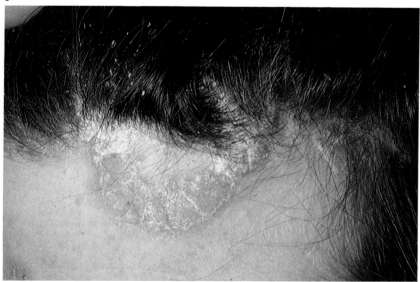

10

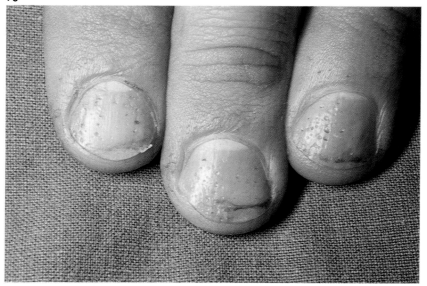

11 *Psoriasis, fingernails* The distal separation of the nail plate (onycholysis) and the irregular salmon-coloured patch are typical of psoriasis.

12 *Psoriasis, penis* A common site. In the uncircumcised the appearance is that of flexural psoriasis.

13 *Psoriasis, palms* Hard dome-shaped lesions are present. It is important to look for psoriasis elsewhere on the skin. Secondary syphilis can look similar to this **(93)**.

11

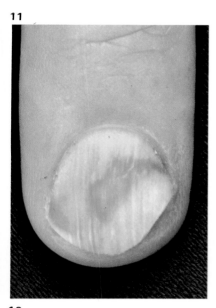

12

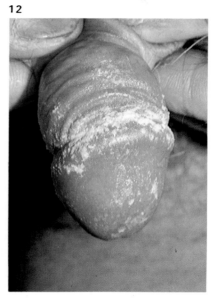

13

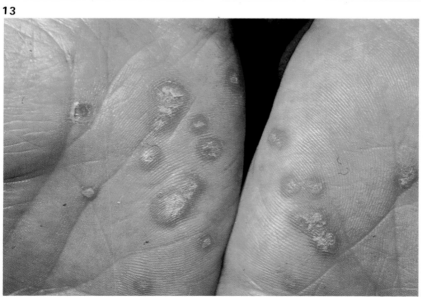

14 *Psoriasis, guttate* The 'spattered' droplet type of psoriasis occurs especially in children and young adults usually following a strepto-coccal throat infection. There is no predilection for the elbows and knees. It usually clears completely in a few months when the infection resolves, but classical psoriasis may develop subsequently.

15 *Psoriasis, erythrodermic* Starting as typical common psoriasis it spreads to involve the whole skin surface. This is one type of erythro-derma (formerly called exfoliative dermatitis), of which there are other causes such as eczema (**70**), reticulosis (**449**) and pityriasis rubra pilaris (**246**).

16 *Psoriasis with psoriatic arthropathy, finger* Psoriatic arthro-pathy resembles rheumatoid arthritis, but serum rheumatoid factor is absent. Distal interphalangeal joint arthritis is characteristic but is by no means always present. Pain and swelling of the finger joints and large joints of the limbs is present in between 5% and 10% of patients with psoriasis and can result in severe disability.

14

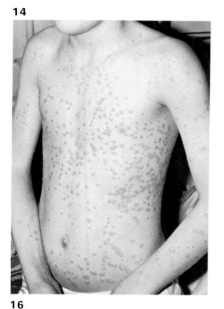

15

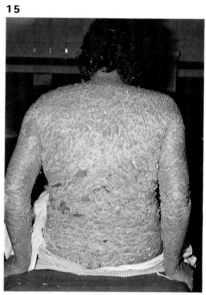

16

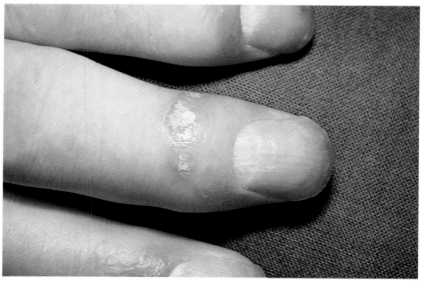

17 *Psoriasis, pustular, palms* The commonest presentation of pustular psoriasis is localised to the palms and soles with no evidence of psoriasis elsewhere. Old pustules leave brownish stains and new ones appear. Sometimes it is part of a generalised pustular psoriasis (**20**). The pus is sterile and this together with the absence of severe tenderness and oedema distinguishes it from infected acute eczema of the palms (**66**).

18 *Psoriasis, pustular, soles* The same observations apply as for the palmar variety. Usually both palms and soles are affected but not always to the same degree.

19 *Psoriasis, pustular, fingertips* Formerly called 'acrodermatitis continua of Hallopeau', this paronychial type affects the extremities of the fingers and toes and may extend proximally. Rarely it may progress to generalised pustular psoriasis with a bad prognosis. The nails tend to be shed at an early stage.

17

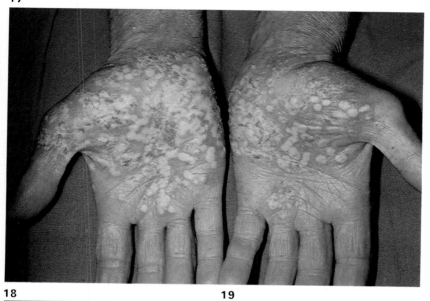

18

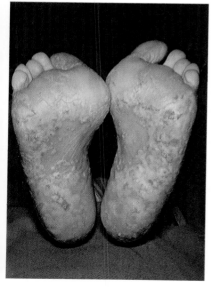

19

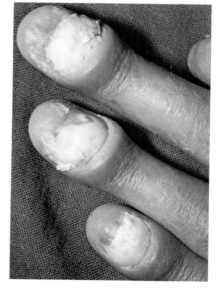

20 *Generalised pustular psoriasis (von Zumbusch)* The patient is severely ill with high fever and prostration. A polymorph leukocytosis of up to 30,000 is present, and there is low serum calcium and steatorrhoea. Widespread crops of superficial pustules appear from day to day on a bright red background. It can be precipitated by systemic corticosteriods. Untreated, this form of psoriasis is not infrequently fatal. When it appears during pregnancy it has been called 'impetigo herpetiformis'.

21 *Psoriasis, tongue* This very rare phenomenon occurs only in generalised pustular psoriasis. Its severity varies in direct proportion to the skin lesions. The appearance is similar to that of 'geographical tongue' **(275)**.

20

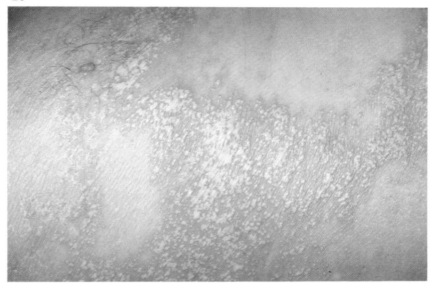

21

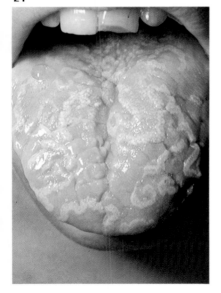

DERMATITIS/ECZEMA

The terms dermatitis and eczema are best regarded as synonymous. To emphasize this point the designation dermatitis/eczema will often appear although normally only one word is used. It refers to a type of inflammation of the skin which has characteristic features both in clinical signs and on microscopy. It may be acute, subacute or chronic.

The *acute* form is red and swollen with papules, vesicles, exudation, serous crusting, and scaling.

The *chronic* form is red, scaly, thickened, dry and sometimes fissured.

The *subacute* form is intermediate between acute and chronic.

No classification of dermatitis/eczema is entirely satisfactory but there is some advantage to consider three categories : those of more or less **'known' cause** ; well-defined morphological and clinical patterns of **unknown cause** ; and those which are **unclassified** pending further elucidation by the natural history of the condition or by investigation.

'KNOWN' CAUSES

Contact dermatitis, irritant, (22–26) Results from excessive exposure to skin irritants, e.g. detergents, soaps, alkalis, solvents.

Contact dermatitis, allergic, (27–41) The individual is specifically sensitized to a particular low molecular weight chemical, e.g. nickel, dichromate, rubber chemicals, organic dyes, topically applied anti-biotics and other medicaments, and a wide range of chemicals used in industrial and domestic life. Positive diagnosis is by patch test (**38–41**).

Gravitational (stasis, varicose), (42–43) Affects the lower legs as a sequel to increased venous pressure, e.g. from incompetent perforat-ing and varicose veins or deep vein thrombosis. It is often complicated by allergic contact dermatitis to a medicament (**35**), by ulceration (**372**), and by spread to other areas ('secondary spread'), (**69**).

Associated with infection & infestation (44) As a complication of bacterial and fungal infections and especially parasitic infestations, e.g. scabies (**169**) and pediculosis (**44**).

Light-induced (45) On the face, backs of hands, and other exposed areas with relation to sun exposure. Not common but may follow drug ingestion (e.g. phenothazine derivatives, tetracyclines, sulphonamides and sulphonyl-urea hypoglycaemic agents) or topical application of photosensitizing chemicals.

Malabsorption & nutritional (46) Rare.   **Drug** Rare.

UNKNOWN CAUSES

Atopic (47–49) Part of the eczema, asthma, hay fever syndrome. The commonest form of infantile eczema. Affects face, neck and distal flexures, i.e. elbow, wrist and knee flexures.

Seborrhoeic (50–56) Manifested by dandruff, itchy scalp, blepharitis, red scaly patches in naso-labial folds and on ears and neck. Patches on presternal area and interscapular region are common. It is sometimes most marked in the major folds, i.e. the groins and axillae.

Lichen simplex (neurodermatitis), (57–60) Thickened pigmented patches at sites easily accessible to scratching. Worse at times of stress. Common sites, nape in women, just below back of elbow, at side of knee or ankle.

Discoid (nummular), (61–63) Assumes a scattered symmetrical coin-shaped pattern.

Palm & sole, *acute* **(64–66)** Recurrent symmetrical itchy blisters on palms and soles ('pompholyx'). Secondary infection is common. *Chronic* **(67)** Symmetrical, dry, hyperkeratotic, thickened, fissured palms and soles.

'Secondary spread' (68, 69) A patch of eczema anywhere may be complicated by a symmetrical widespread dermatitis which may be discoid or confluent. It often accompanies gravitational eczema and acute palm and sole eczema.

Erythrodermic eczema (70) Generalised dermatitis/eczema with no normal skin areas remaining, which is not generalised psoriasis, reticulosis or other individual dermatosis.

UNCLASSIFIED (71, 72)

Many eczematous eruptions do not fit conveniently into either the unknown or known categories. Their classification must be regarded as pending until investigation is complete.

22 *Irritant contact dermatitis, hand* This shows typical changes of dermatitis : redness, scaling, weeping, vesiculation, hyperkeratosis and fissuring. This pattern is produced by contact with irritants such as strong detergents, soaps, alkalis and solvents. A similar reaction tends to occur under wedding rings. It is *not* an allergic reaction.

23 *Irritant contact dermatitis, lip licking* This child readily demonstrated her technique of lip licking which has produced the lesions, a marginated perioral zone of dry scaly inflammation. It is not uncommon in children but parents will not always accept that lip licking is the cause.

24 *Irritant contact dermatitis, chest* The patient washed her bra using strong bleach and rinsing was incomplete.

22

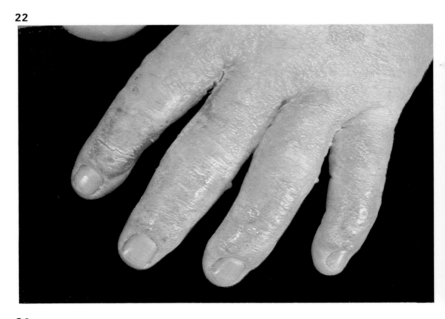

23

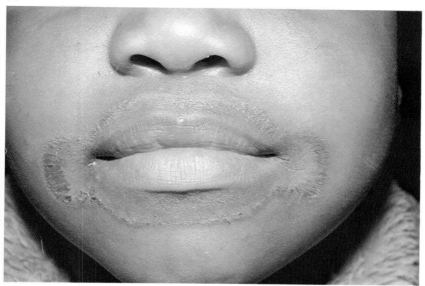

24

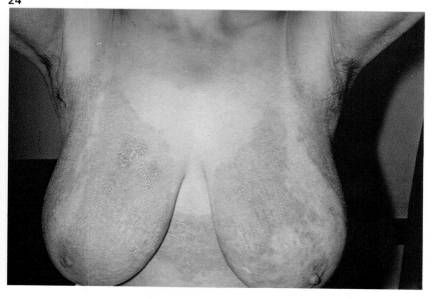

25 *Eczema, irritant contact ('eczéma craquelé') of shin* Over-enthusiastic washing leads to drying and cracking of the stratum corneum. Not infrequently seen in hospital wards, the shins are usually the first to be affected. Avoidance of soap and application of a simple ointment lead to rapid cure.

26 *Eczema, irritant contact ('eczéma craquelé') of shin, close-up* Linear cracking of the stratum corneum produces a mild inflammation.

27 *Allergic contact dermatitis, hair dye* The margins of the scalp are usually most affected. The allergen is paraphenylenediamine (or related chemical), a constituent of many dark dyes. The patient may have used the preparation without ill effects for months or years before sensitization occurs, but once it does each application will lead to dermatitis within 24 – 48 hours.

25

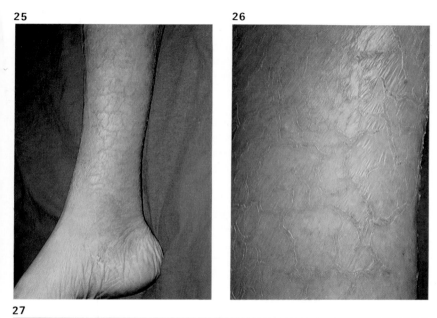

26

27

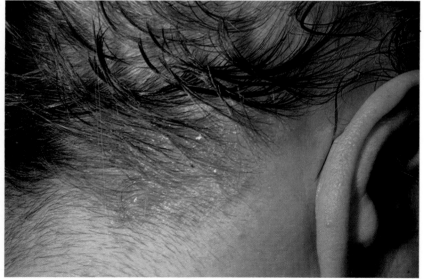

28 *Allergic contact dermatitis, nickel* Patients sensitive to nickel will produce lesions under white metal jewellery or fastenings, e.g. earrings, necklace and bra clips, watch bands and zips. A watch band clasp was responsible in the patient shown. Patch test positive to 5% nickel sulphate solution.

29 *Allergic contact dermatitis, adhesive plaster* The patient was sensitive to colophony resin in adhesive plaster. Blistering is prominent in this case. Patients should be asked about previous adhesive plaster reactions before it is applied. Patch test positive to 20% colophony in soft paraffin.

30 *Allergic contact dermatitis, perfume* Sensitization can occur to one of the essential oils or a 'fixative' (e.g. balsam of Peru) in the perfume.

28

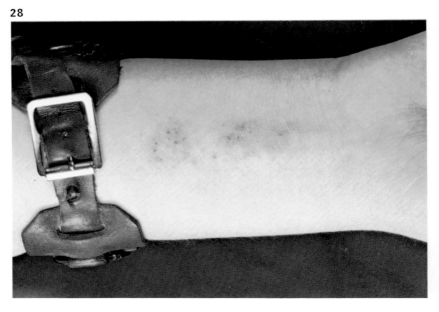

29

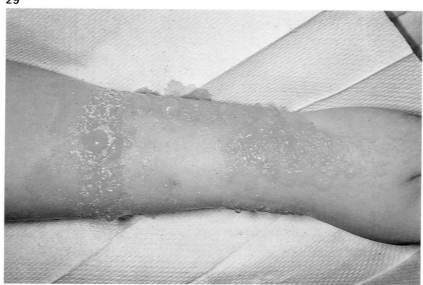

30

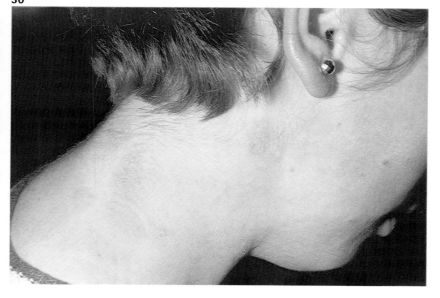

31 *Allergic contact dermatitis, nail varnish* The fingers are not affected due to care of application of the varnish but small quantities rub off on the eyelids, face, neck or other areas when they are touched with the fingernails and dermatitis results. Patch test positive. The allergen is an aryl sulphonamide formaldehyde resin.

32 *Allergic contact dermatitis, shoes* The patient did not realize she was sensitive to rubber chemicals in the soles of her shoes. The chemicals (usually mercaptobenzothiazole or tetramethylthiuramdisulphide) are absorbed through to the foot. The pressure points of the sole are the worst affected, and the proximal parts of the toes and the toe-webs are clear. This condition is often misdiagnosed as fungal infection. The treatment is to wear rubber-free footwear. Patch test positive to 1% chemical. The above chemicals are often present in garments containing rubber or rubber substitutes and may give rise to dermatitis at sites of contact.

31

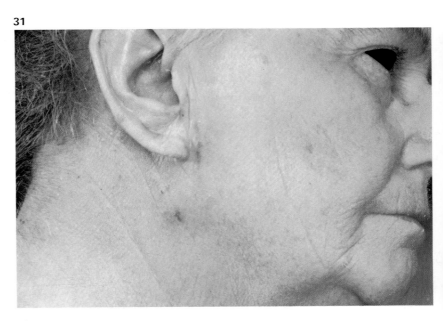

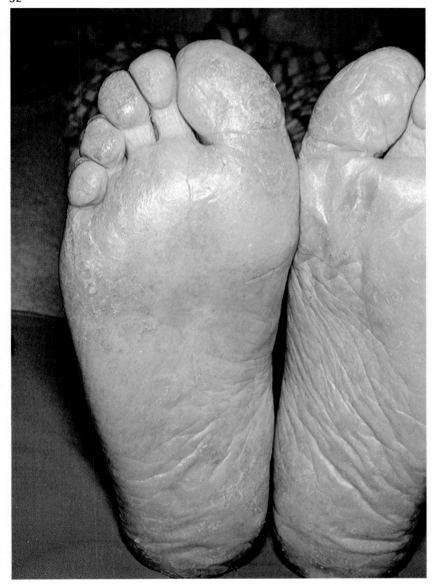

33 *Allergic contact dermatitis, face* The patient became sensitive to benzylperoxide in a therapeutic face cream. Facial eczema is often very oedematous, especially on the eyelids, and is often misdiagnosed as erysipelas (**86**). Dermatitis is pruritic, an important diagnostic symptom. The white appearance is due to calamine lotion which is not the most cosmetic of treatments for the face.

34 *Allergic contact dermatitis, chrysanthemum* In addition to lesions on the upper limbs, as shown here, an acute dermatitis of the face may be produced. Examples of plants which can cause allergic contact dermatitis are primula, chrysanthemum, tulip and garlic. In the United States the commonest plant dermatitis is the result of Rhus (poison ivy, poison oak) sensitivity where it presents as streaks and patches of dermatitis, often with blisters.

35 *Allergic contact dermatitis to medicated tulle* The patient has mild gravitational ulceration. The tulle dressing contained soframycin to which she had become sensitive. Soframycin often cross-reacts with neomycin, which is a fairly common sensitizer.

33

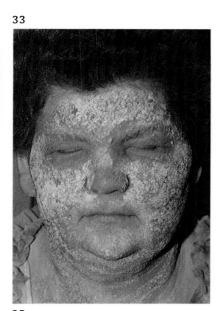

34

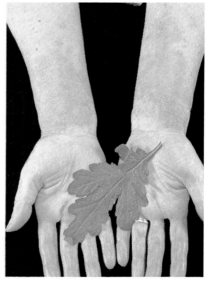

35

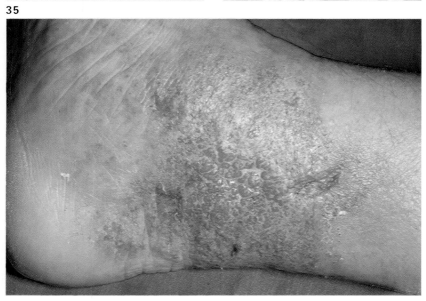

36 *Berloque dermatitis, neck and chest* This lesion is caused by perfume containing a *psoralen*, i.e. a chemical which renders the skin sensitive to light at the site of application. The result is inflammation at the site with subsequent post-inflammatory hyperpigmentation. The streaky pattern is typical. The psoralen in perfume is usually bergamot oil

37 *Tattoo, reaction to red pigment* The patient had an allergic reaction to mercury in the cinnebar pigment.

38 *Patch testing, preparation* To confirm the diagnosis of allergic contact dermatitis, patch testing with appropriate concentrations of a series of common sensitizers is carried out. The chemicals are dissolved in water or in soft paraffin ointment and are applied in sequence to patch test dressings as shown. In addition to the group of chemicals used for all such patients other sensitizers can be tested as suggested by the patient's history, occupation or hobbies. It is most important that the correct concentration of the test substance is used for patch testing (information on this is to be found in dermatological text books and monographs). Some known sensitizers are irritant in high concentration and false-positive reactions can occur.

36

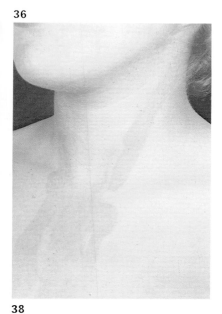

37

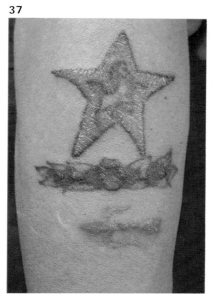

38

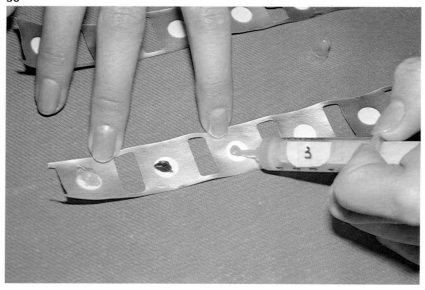

39 & 40 *Patch testing, application* Patch test dressings treated with the desired sequence of chemicals are placed in position on the back (or other convenient part of the skin surface) and are occluded with waterproof adhesive plaster. If the patient is known to be sensitive to the usual adhesive plaster, plastic or paper adhesive tape is used. The tests are left undisturbed for 48 – 72 hours.

41 *Patch testing, results* At the end of 48 – 72 hours the test dressings are discarded and test sites are inspected for inflammation. Positive tests will be pruritic and show erythema and oedema with variable degrees of vesiculation and exudation. A positive patch test indicates allergic sensitivity to the chemical applied. Positive results are recorded and correlated with the patient's eruption and history to determine their exact relevance to the dermatitis under investigation. Shown here are positive patch test reactions to two concentrations of dinitrochloro-benzene (DNCB), a potent sensitizer, with a negative control patch (C).

39

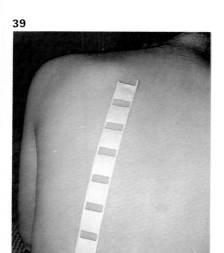

40

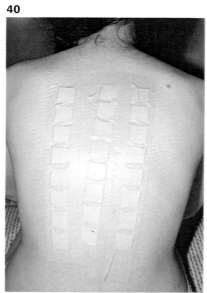

41

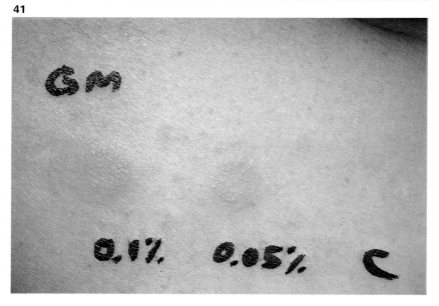

GM

0.1%   0.05%   C

42 *Dermatitis, gravitational (stasis, varicose), ankle* This very common form of eczema is usually associated with varicose or incompetent perforating veins of the leg. It is often complicated by oedema, infection, ulceration, allergic contact sensitization to topical medicaments and secondary spread of eczema to the face and other area. The common allergens are lanolin, antibiotics, antibacterial agents and preservatives.

43 *Dermatitis, gravitational (stasis, varicose), acute-on-chronic* Sudden exacerbation of chronic gravitational dermatitis suggests infection or allergic contact sensitization to a medicament.

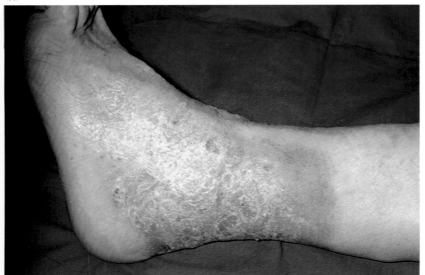

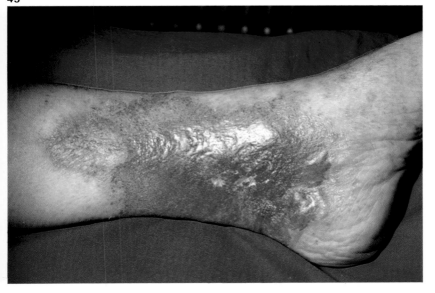

44 *Dermatitis/eczema, associated with infestation* The patient had widespread excoriated chronic eczema. Pediculosis corporis was confirmed by finding lice and eggs in the seams of his clothing (**173**). Scabies may also produce widespread eczema (**169**).

45 *Dermatitis/eczema, light-induced, face* The patient developed an eczematous eruption in sunlight-exposed areas (i.e. the face and backs of the hands). This distribution, where the covered areas are spared, should always raise the suspicion of light sensitivity (see section on light-induced dermatoses).

46 *Eczema due to malabsorption* The patient had patchy eczema and hyperpigmentation associated with steatorrhoea. Lesions show no specific features and the association with malabsorption is not common. The eruption cleared after the patient started a gluten-free diet.

44

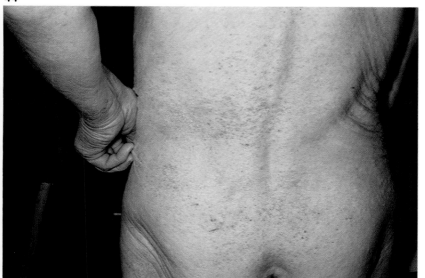

45

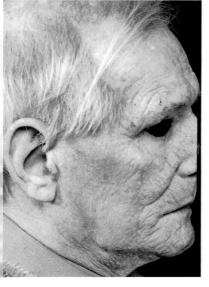

46

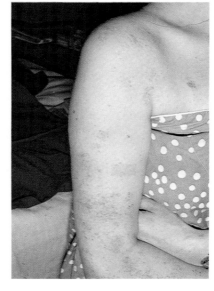

47 & 48 *Atopic dermatitis, elbow, wrist and knee flexures* This type of dermatitis is often associated with a personal and/or family history of asthma and hay fever. Common in infants and children it tends to settle in the distal flexures (wrist and ankle flexures, elbow and knee flexures) during early childhood. It is the commonest type of so-called 'Infantile eczema'. Lesions are also present on the face and neck. They are very pruritic and when scratched become excoriated and lichenified. The whole skin is usually very dry (atopic xerosis). Atopic dermatitis usually clears by puberty, but may persist for several decades. In dark-skinned patients (**47**) chronic eczema shows inflammatory hyper-pigmentation.

47

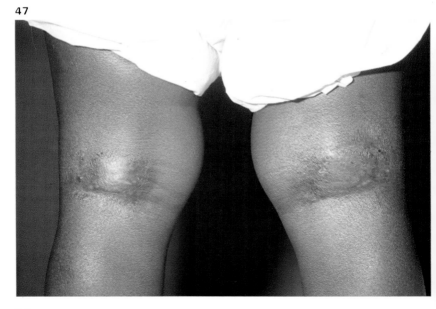

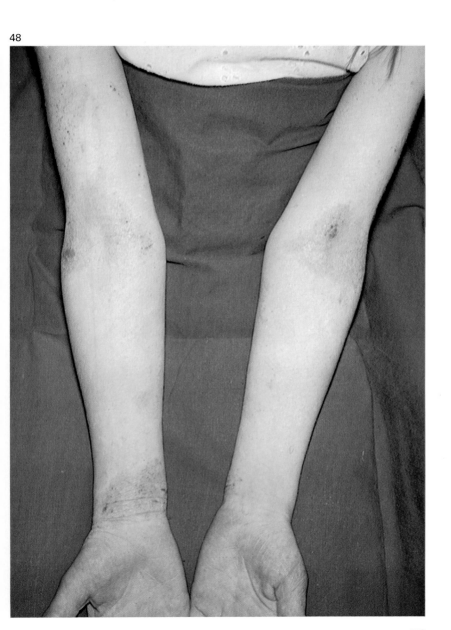

49 *Atopic dermatitis, perioral* The area around the mouth is commonly involved. The vermillion of the lips is dry and scaly. The area adjacent to the centre of the upper lip is often the last to clear. Sometimes in this disorder the whole face is of a uniform pale pink colour with dryness and fine scaling.

50 & 51 *'Seborrhoeic' dermatitis, face, axillae and groins* The term 'seborrhoeic' is anachronistic and not related to aetiology. It is usually used for an eczematous pattern of unknown cause appearing in the axillae and groins, on the scalp, face, neck and ears, and in presternal and interscapular regions. Secondary bacterial infection may occur.

49

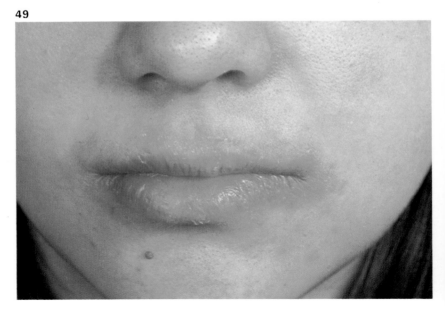

50

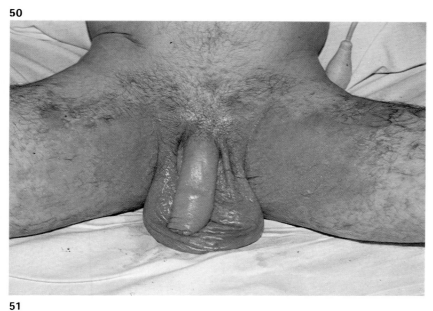

51

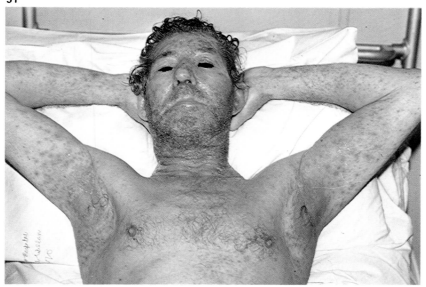

52 *'Seborrhoeic' dermatitis, infantile* The 'napkin (diaper) eruption' is common in infants. It is not usually related to atopic dermatitis and clears within a few weeks with appropriate treatment. It is sometimes called 'napkin psoriasis' but its connection with common psoriasis is uncertain. There are some who regard it as due to candida infection or milk allergy, but conclusive evidence is lacking.

53 *'Seborrhoeic' dermatitis, infantile* More severe napkin (diaper) eruption in a child of Caribbean origin.

54 *Ammoniacal dermatitis, infantile* This napkin (diaper) eruption has become ulcerative due to very poor hygiene. If wet napkins are left in position urine decomposition liberates ammonia which is a skin irritant.

52

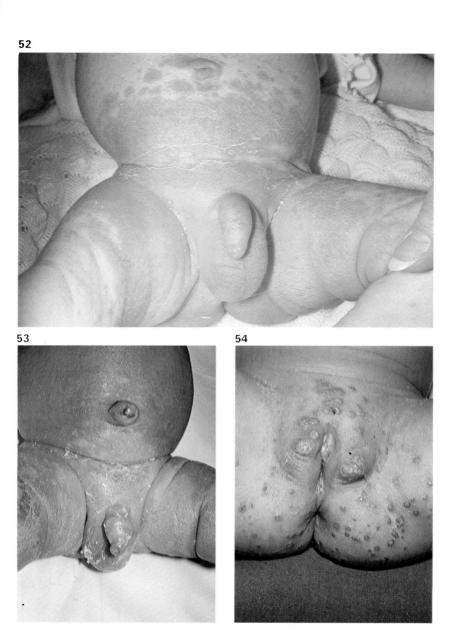

53

54

55 *'Seborrhoeic' dermatitis, infantile, scalp and forehead lesions*
Thick greasy scales in the scalp ('cradle cap') and red scaly patches on
the head and neck are often seen in association with napkin (diaper)
eruption.

56 *'Seborrhoeic' dermatitis 'seborrhoeide'* Adults with dandruff
sometimes develop symmetrical brownish scaly patches on the neck and
shoulders. Treating the scalp usually clears the rash.

57 *Lichen simplex ('localised neurodermatitis'), nape of neck*
Tense individuals who scratch a particular area of skin when under stress
often develop a single patch of lichenified eczema. The nape pattern is
virtually seen only in women. It is a thickened plaque with exaggerated
skin markings thrown up in relief.

58 *Lichen simplex, scrotum* A fissured, thickened (lichenified)
eczema is shown. This is sometimes misdiagnosed as a fungal infection.
Mycological examination of skin scrapings is necessary.

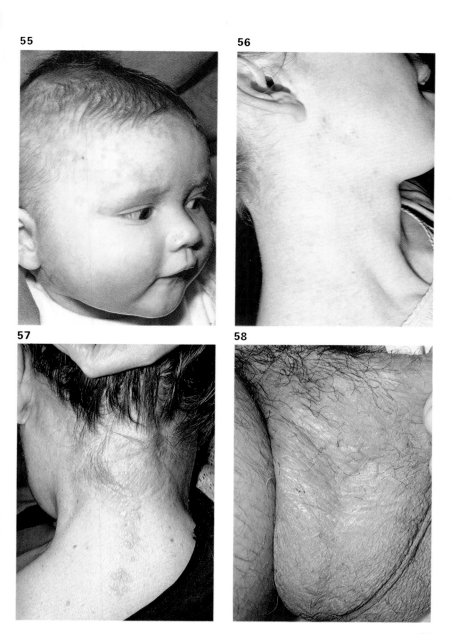

59 *Lichen simplex ('localised neurodermatitis'), lateral shin*
The patient was a telephonist who scratched his left leg with his left
hand when the switchboard became busy. A differential diagnosis would
be hypertrophic lichen planus (**191**).

60 *Lichen simplex, perianal* This is one type of lesion which causes
pruritus ani and it tends to occur in individuals with an 'obsessional' per-
sonality. Pruritus ani may however be due to other causes ; e.g. discharge
from haemorrhoids, allergic contact dermatitis to constituents of topical
applications or suppositories, anal fissures, and excessive sweating.

59

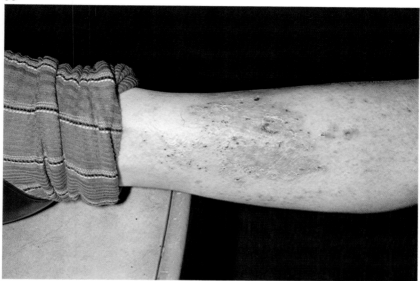

60

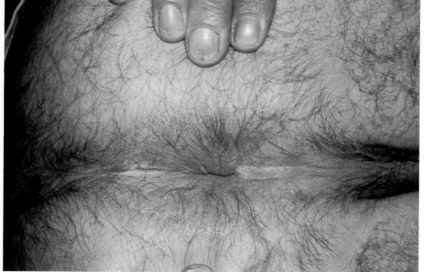

61, 62 & 63 *Discoid eczema (nummular dermatitis), hand, arms and legs* Fairly symmetrical, small round coin-shaped plaques of eczema appear on the limbs, usually on extensor surfaces. Serous crusting is common. Young adults are frequently affected. It is sometimes part of a secondary spread from eczema elsewhere (see **68**) but usually no cause is found. It is not related to atopic eczema.

61

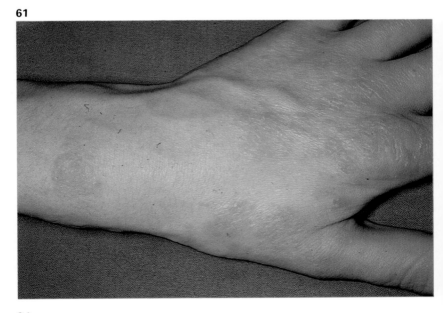

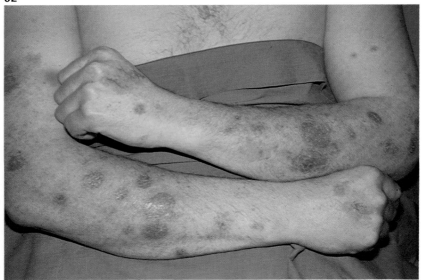

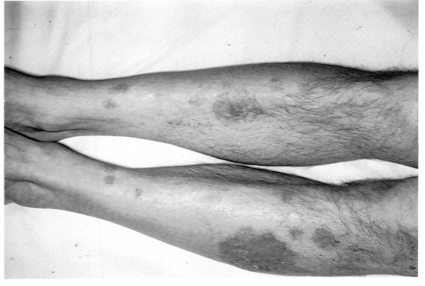

64 *Palm and sole eczema, acute vesicular ('pompholyx'), palms*
A fairly common pattern of eczema which can be recurrent. Usually no
cause is demonstrable but this pattern can be due to trichophytin sensitivity and associated with fungal infection of the feet. Sometimes the
epidermal vesicles resemble sago grains which can only be seen on close
inspection. This patient's blisters were unusually large.

65 *Palm and sole eczema, acute vesicular, soles* The soles were
intensely pruritic. There was no evidence of fungal infection or of allergic
contact eczema.

66 *Palm and sole eczema, acute infected, palm* Secondary infection in acute vesicular eczema of the palms is a common complication. Pus forms in the blisters and the hands are red, swollen and very
painful. Lymphangitis and fever may be present. Staphylococci or strep-
tococci are grown from swabs of the pus.

64

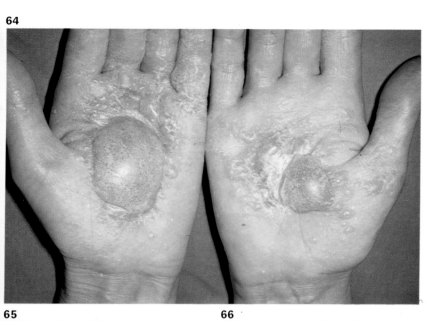

65

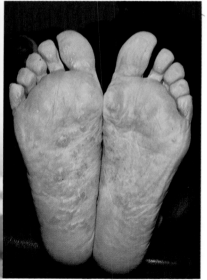

66

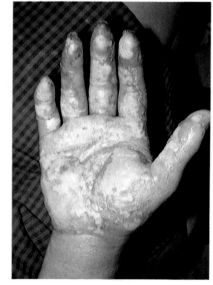

67 *Palm and sole eczema, chronic hyperkeratotic and fissured*
This chronic condition may follow on from the acute form or may start in this way. The stratum corneum is thick, dry and brittle so that hand movements result in painful cracks. Avoidance of soap, and a greasy application are indicated.

68 *Dermatitis/eczema, secondary spread* Eczema can spread from the primary site either locally or to give a widespread symmetrical eruption. The patient's primary lesion was on the left wrist and was due to allergic contact dermatitis from a watch strap, which contained nickel.

69 *Dermatitis/eczema, secondary spread, face* The patient presented complaining of the face eruption only. When she undressed it was found that she had an acute-on-chronic gravitational eczema of the left ankle which was the primary lesion. This situation is by no means uncommon and a full examination of the skin is mandatory.

70 *Erythrodermic eczema (exfoliative dermatitis)* Almost any variety of eczema if neglected or treated inappropriately can spread to involve the whole skin surface. Drug eruptions, especially those due to heavy metals, sometimes take this form.

67

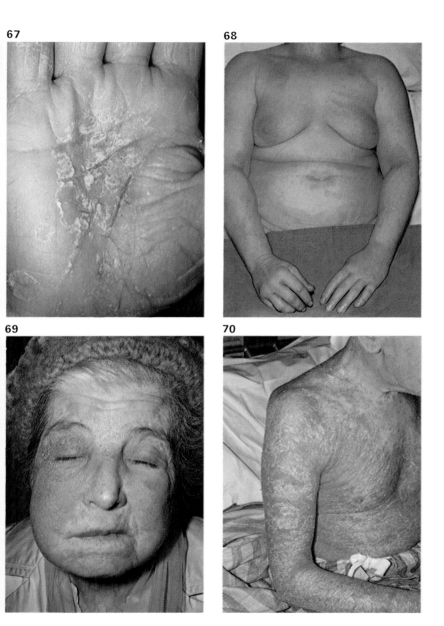

68

69

70

71 *Dermatitis/eczema, unclassified, exfoliative cheilitis* The pattern of eczema in a particular patient may defy classification. Unclassified eczema requires investigation at least to the extent of scraping for fungus and patch testing. No cause was found for this eruption of the lips.

72 *Dermatitis/eczema, unclassified, unilateral nipple* Unilateral eczema of the nipple must be suspected of being Paget's disease of the nipple (intra-duct carcinoma, **331**) until proven otherwise by skin biopsy. In this patient the histology showed only eczema and the condition cleared with treatment.

71

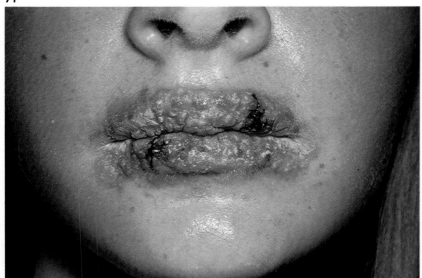

72

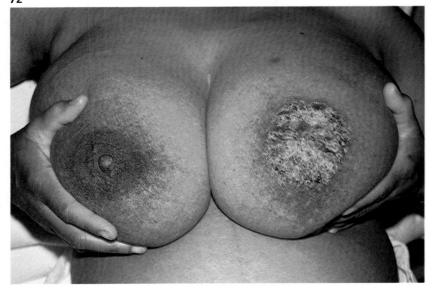

INFECTIONS AND INFESTATIONS

Correct diagnosis of skin infections and infestations is of great importance since curative therapy by specific topical or systemic medicaments is usually readily available, and they may be made worse by corticosteroids.

Bacterial infections
folliculitis **73**
sycosis barbae **74**
furuncle **75, 76**
stye **77**
impetigo contagiosa **78–82**
ecthyma **83**
lymphangitis & cellulitis **84**
erysipelas **85, 86**
septicaemia **87**
dental sinus **88**
syphilis **89–99**
tuberculosis **100–104**
leprosy **105–108**
erythrasma **137, 138**

Protozoal infection
leishmaniasis **109**

Fungal infections
tinea capitis **110, 111**
tinea corporis **112–122**

Yeast infections
candidiasis **123–132**
pityriasis versicolor **133–136**

Viral infections
viral warts **139–147**
molluscum contagiosum **148–150**
herpes simplex **151–156**
vaccinia **157–159**
herpes zoster **160–162**

possible viral infections
pityriasis rosea **163–166**
Gianotti-Crosti syndrome **167**

Infestations
scabies **168–172**
pediculosis **173–178**
insect bites **179, 180**
creeping eruption **181**

73 *Folliculitis* Hair follicles in adults are liable to become infected with staphylococci. Hairy areas subject to moistness and friction are particularly at risk (e.g. axillae and the back of the neck under the collar). Folliculitis may arise as a complication following the application of a corticosteroid ointment. It starts as a red spot around the follicular orifice, and develops into a superficial pustule.

74 *Folliculitis, sycosis barbae* Shaving in men can spread staphylococcal infection from follicle to follicle. The example shown is relatively mild. Very severe forms, common in the past, are now rarely seen.

73

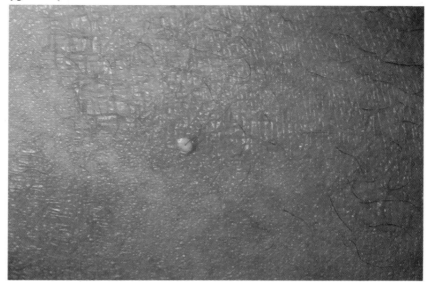

74

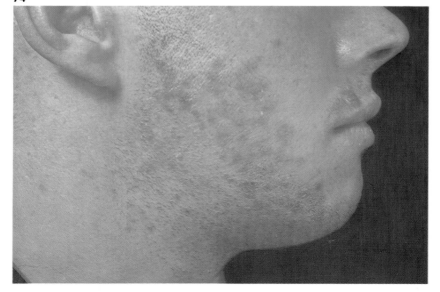

75 *Furuncle (boil)*   If the staphylococcal infection of a hair follicle extends throughout its length to be accompanied by intense inflammation and suppuration it is called a furuncle. If several adjacent hair follicles are involved with confluent inflammation it is called a 'carbuncle'. These lesions are very painful.

76 *Furunculosis, axilla*   Furunculosis can be a presenting sign of diabetes mellitus and the urine should be tested for sugar.

77 *Stye (hordeolum), lower eyelid*   A stye is a boil in an eyelash follicle. Most cases carry pathogenic staphylococci in the anterior nares as well as in the lesion and both require treatment with an antibiotic or antibacterial ointment.

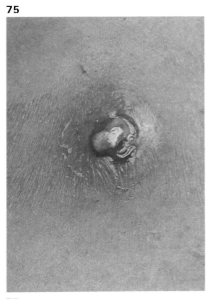

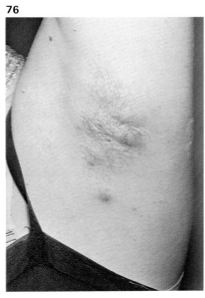

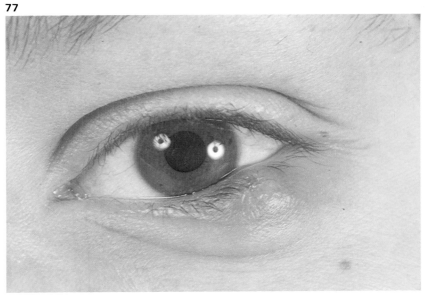

78 *Impetigo contagiosa, face* This is a spreading staphylococcal or streptococcal infection of the epidermis. It is common in children and often spreads from the nostrils which form a reservoir of bacteria for infection. Scratching and personal contact spread the infection, and other members of the family are frequently affected. The condition is common during the summer months. In tropical countries lesions may be widespread and severe and epidemics occur. It clears rapidly with antibiotic ointment. When the predominant organism is the streptococcus, impetigo can be followed by acute glomerulonephritis.

79 *Impetigo contagiosa, circinate lesions, chin*

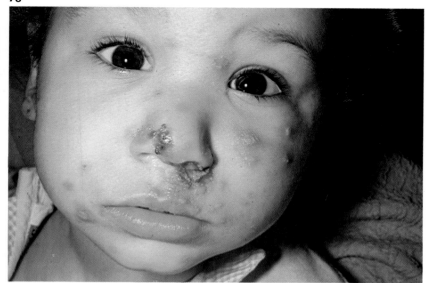

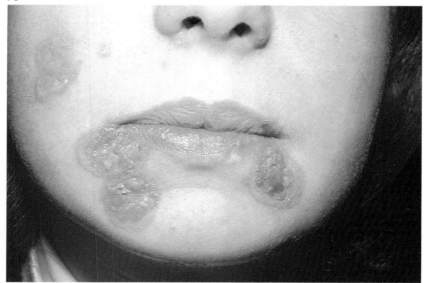

80 *Impetigo contagiosa, face* The superficial nature of the infection and characteristic honey-coloured serous crusting are apparent. Eczema and herpes simplex lesions can become infected and 'impetiginized'.

81 *Impetigo contagiosa* If the infection is of low-grade severity thick serous crusts may form, as on this girl's face.

82 *Bullous impetigo contagiosa, trunk* If the infection spreads rapidly in a young child the stratum corneum is raised to become the roof of a superficial blister, and it ruptures to form an erosion. Blisters and erosions are seen here on the trunk of a child.

83 *Ecthyma* Bacterial infections can produce small, deep, crusted ulcers which eventually heal with scarring. This occurs particularly in the malnourished.

80

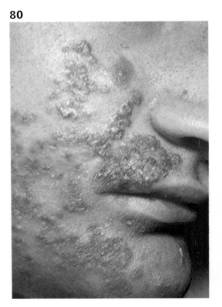

81

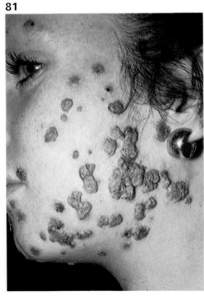

82

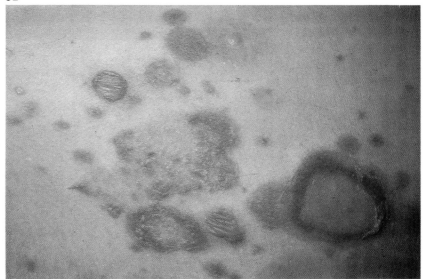

83

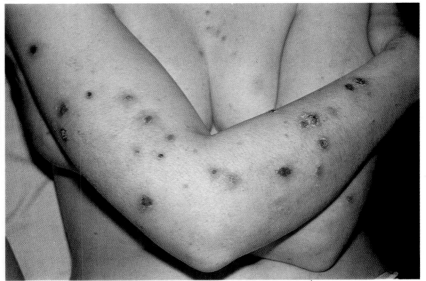

84 *Lymphangitis and cellulitis*   Tender red streaks up the arm or leg are due to streptococcal infection in lymphatic vessels draining an infected extremity. Common causes are infected eczema of the hands and feet and fungal infection of the toe-webs with fissuring. Enlarged tender lymph nodes in the axillae or groin may be found and high fever with rigors can be associated features. A differential diagnosis is thrombophlebitis.

85 *Erysipelas, leg*   The leg is the most common site for this infection. Purpura is common in inflammatory lesions of the legs, whatever the cause.

86 *Erysipelas, face*   An acute streptococcal infection with tender erythema and oedema. Recurrent episodes can be associated with increasing lymphoedema.

84

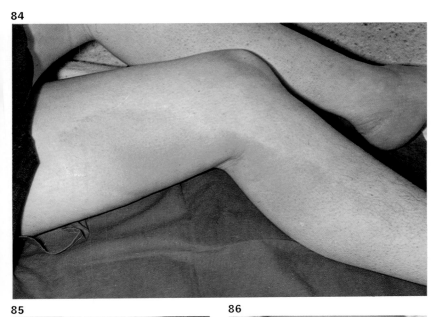

85

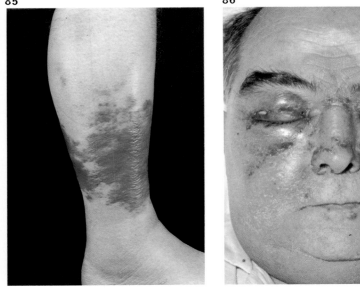

86

87 *Septicaemia* The patient developed extremely tender skin lesions with fever and a positive blood culture following hysterectomy. Individual lesions resemble erythema multiforme (see **349**), but they differ in that they are larger, very tender and irregularly distributed.

88 *Dental sinus* A dental apical abscess can open on the skin anywhere on the face and jaw area to produce a chronic granulating sinus. A typical lesion is shown. Extraction of the infected tooth is curative.

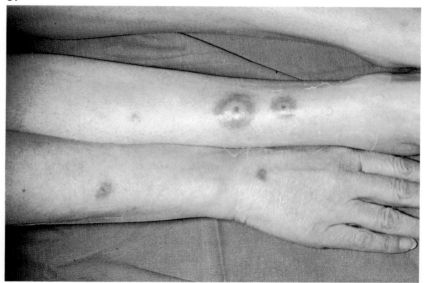

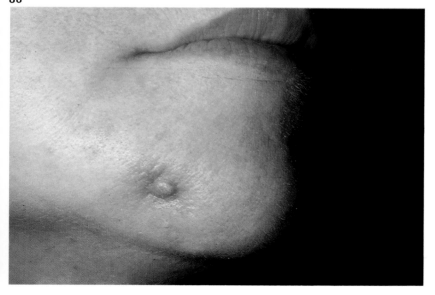

89 *Syphilis, secondary, 'roseola syphilide'* There is a symmetrical profuse eruption of subtle pink macules and barely raised papules at all stages of development. Examination in daylight is usually necessary to see this eruption, it can be completely missed in artificial light. The papular element is best seen here on the patient's left side where the light strikes it obliquely. Patients with secondary syphilis usually feel generally unwell ; this can be a helpful diagnostic point in association with other evidence. Pruritus is minimal or absent.

90 *Syphilis, secondary* This is at a later stage of development than in **89**. Scattered papules are seen. The patient felt unwell and had a generalised lymphadenopathy.

89

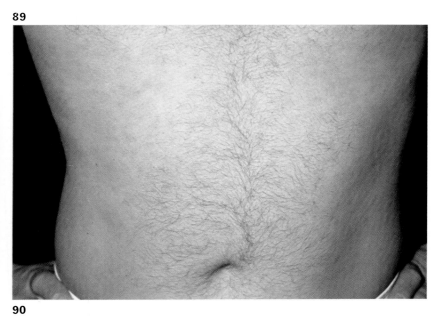

90

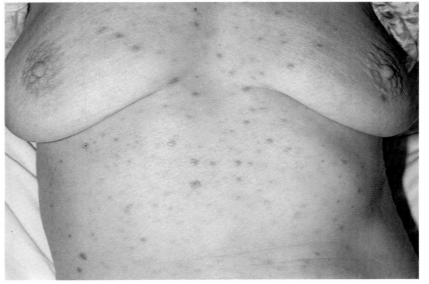

91 *Syphilis, secondary, trunk* This florid eruption resembled a 'toxic' erythema (see **344**).

92 *Syphilis, secondary* Individual papules may resemble psoriasis. The whole skin surface and mucous membranes must be examined. Serology is always strongly positive in secondary lues.

93 *Secondary syphilis, palms* Smooth-topped or scaly symmetrical, brownish papules on the palms and soles are a feature of late secondary syphilis. Patchy loss of scalp hair may also be found.

91

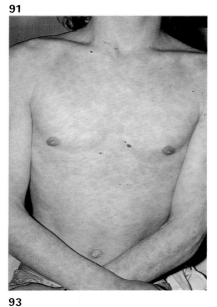

92

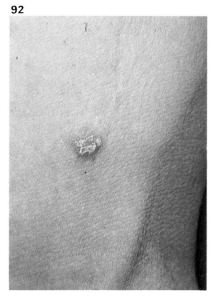

93

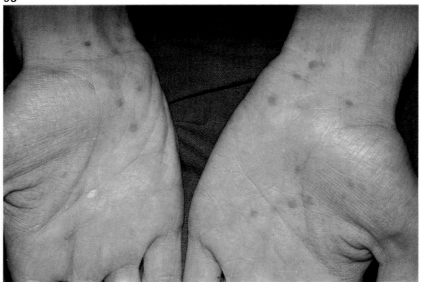

94 *Secondary syphilis, soles* These papules are similar to those on the palms.

95 *Secondary syphilis, mucous patches, mouth* Two mucous patches are present to the left of the tip of the tongue. They are superficial erosions covered by a thin white slough. The whitish membrane is easily scraped off. They can arise on any part of the tongue or oral mucosa and are usually painless. Treponemes abound in these lesions.

96 *Secondary syphilis, condylomata lata* Syphilitic raised papules ('warts') occur in the perineum or in any moist intertriginous site. These lesions teem with spirochaetes, they are therefore dark-ground positive and highly contagious. They must be distinguished from viral warts in this area, i.e. condylomata acuminata (**144**).

94

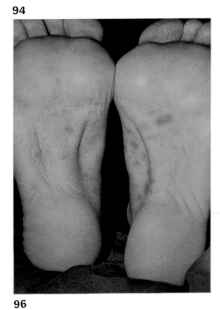

95

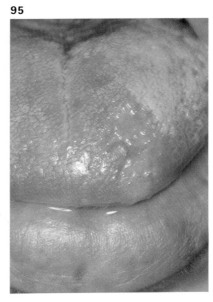

96

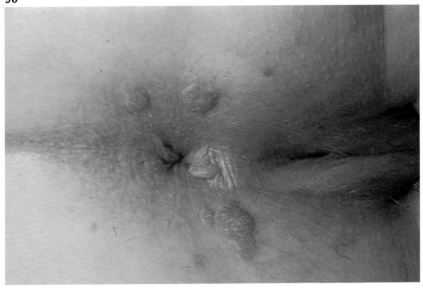

97 *Syphilis, gumma* Note central clearing and extending nodular margin. The lesion was symptomless.

98 *Syphilis, gumma of back* A less florid example than in **97**, but central clearing, peripheral extension and nodulation are still obvious.

99 *Syphilis, ulcerated gumma of calf* The blood Wasserman reaction, or other serological test for syphilis, is an essential investigation in all chronic leg ulcers.

97

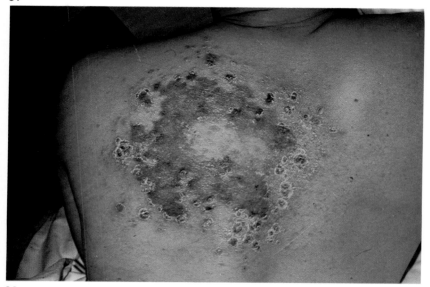

98

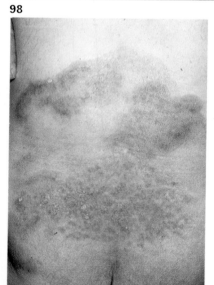

99

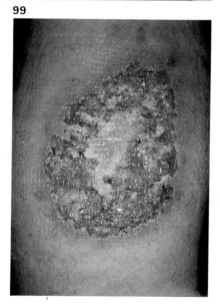

100 *Lupus vulgaris, cheek* Cutaneous tuberculosis in a patient with a strongly positive tuberculin test. The lesion had been growing untreated for nearly 20 years. It was symptomless. It consisted of clusters of raised brownish-red papules. Atrophy and scarring also occur, particularly after treatment.

101 *Lupus vulgaris, diascopy* Individual granulomatous tubercles are shown up by pressing a microscope slide or transparent spatula over the lesion. The procedure squeezes out the blood from the lesion and small translucent brownish papules are seen. They are sometimes called 'apple jelly' nodules.

100

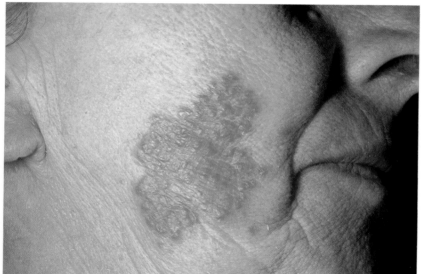

101

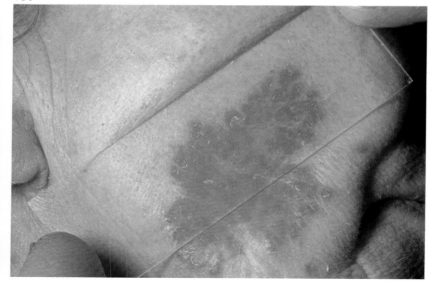

LOTRISONE®
brand of clotrimazole and betamethasone dipropionate
Cream, USP

For Dermatologic Use Only– Not for Ophthalmic Use

DESCRIPTION LOTRISONE Cream contains a combination of clotrimazole, USP, a synthetic antifungal agent, and betamethasone dipropionate, USP, a synthetic corticosteroid, for dermatologic use.

Chemically, clotrimazole is 1-(o-Chloro-α,α-diphenyl benzyl) imidazole, with the empirical formula $C_{22}H_{17}ClN_2$, a molecular weight of 344.8, and the following structural formula:

Clotrimazole is an odorless, white crystalline powder, insoluble in water and soluble in ethanol.

Betamethasone dipropionate has the chemical name 9-Fluoro-11β, 17,21-trihydroxy-16β-methylpregna-1, 4-diene-3,20-dione 17,21-dipropionate, with the empirical formula $C_{28}H_{37}FO_7$, a molecular weight of 504.6, and the following structural formula:

Betamethasone dipropionate is a white to creamy white, odorless crystalline powder, insoluble in water.

Each gram of LOTRISONE Cream contains 10.0 mg clotrimazole, USP, and 0.64 mg betamethasone dipropionate, USP (equivalent to 0.5 mg betamethasone), in a hydrophilic emollient cream consisting of purified water, mineral oil, white petrolatum, cetearyl alcohol, ceteareth-30, propylene glycol, sodium phosphate monobasic, and phosphoric acid; benzyl alcohol as preservative.

LOTRISONE is a smooth, uniform, white to off-white cream.

CLINICAL PHARMACOLOGY

Clotrimazole

Clotrimazole is a broad-spectrum, antifungal agent that is used for the treatment of dermal infections caused by various species of pathogenic dermatophytes, yeasts, and *Malassezia furfur*. The primary action of clotrimazole is against dividing and growing organisms.

In vitro, clotrimazole exhibits fungistatic and fungicidal activity against isolates of *Trichophyton rubrum*, *Trichophyton mentagrophytes*, *Epidermophyton floccosum* and *Microsporum canis*. In general, the *in vitro* activity of clotrimazole corresponds to that of tolnaftate and griseofulvin against the mycelia of dermatophytes (*Trichophyton*, *Microsporum*, and *Epidermophyton*).

In vivo studies in guinea pigs infected with *Trichophyton mentagrophytes* have shown no measurable loss of clotrimazole activity due to combination with betamethasone dipropionate.

Strains of fungi having a natural resistance to clotrimazole have not been reported.

No single-step or multiple-step resistance to clotrimazole has developed during successive passages of *Trichophyton mentagrophytes*.

In studies of the mechanism of action in fungal cultures, the minimum fungicidal concentration of clotrimazole caused leakage of intracellular phosphorous compounds into the ambient medium with concomitant breakdown of cellular nucleic acids, and accelerated potassium efflux. Both of these events began rapidly and extensively after addition of the drug to the cultures.

Clotrimazole appears to be minimally absorbed following topical application to the skin. Six hours after the application of radioactive clotrimazole 1% cream and 1% solution onto intact and acutely inflamed skin, the concentration of clotrimazole varied from 100 mcg/cm3 in the stratum corneum, to 0.5 to 1 mcg/cm3 in the stratum reticulare, and 0.1 mcg/cm3 in the subcutis. No measurable amount of radioactivity ($<$0.001 mcg/mL) was found in the serum within 48 hours after application under occlusive dressing of 0.5 mL of the solution or 0.8 g of the cream.

Betamethasone dipropionate

Betamethasone dipropionate, a corticosteroid, is effective in the treatment of corticosteroid-responsive dermatoses primarily because of its anti-inflammatory, antipruritic, and vasoconstrictive actions. However, while the physiologic, pharmacologic, and clinical effects of corticosteroids are well-known, the exact mechanisms of their actions in each disease are uncertain. Betamethasone dipropionate, a corticosteroid, has been shown to have topical (dermatologic) and systemic pharmacologic and metabolic effects characteristic of this class of drugs.

Pharmacokinetics The extent of percutaneous absorption of topical corticosteroids is determined by many factors including the vehicle, the integrity of the epidermal barrier, and the use of occlusive dressings. (See **DOSAGE AND ADMINISTRATION** section.)

Topical corticosteroids can be absorbed from normal intact skin. Inflammation and/or other disease processes in the skin increase percutaneous absorption. Occlusive dressings substantially increase the percutaneous absorption of topical corticosteroids. (See **DOSAGE AND ADMINISTRATION** section.)

Once absorbed through the skin, topical corticosteroids are handled through pharmacokinetic pathways similar to systemically administered corticosteroids. Corticosteroids are bound to plasma proteins in varying degrees. Corticosteroids are metabolized primarily in the liver and are then excreted by the kidneys. Some of the topical corticosteroids and their metabolites are also excreted into the bile.

Clotrimazole and betamethasone dipropionate

In clinical studies of tinea corporis, tinea cruris, and tinea pedis, patients treated with LOTRISONE Cream showed a better clinical response at the first return visit than patients treated with clotrimazole cream. In tinea corporis and tinea cruris, the patient returned 3 days after starting treatment, and in tinea pedis, after 1 week. Mycological cure rates observed in patients treated with LOTRISONE Cream were as good as or better than in those patients treated with clotrimazole cream.

In these same clinical studies, patients treated with LOTRISONE Cream showed statistically significantly better clinical responses and mycological cure rates when compared with patients treated with betamethasone dipropionate cream.

INDICATIONS AND USAGE LOTRISONE Cream is indicated for the topical treatment of the following dermal infections: tinea pedis, tinea cruris, and tinea corporis due to *Trichophyton rubrum*, *Trichophyton mentagrophytes*, *Epidermophyton floccosum*, and *Microsporum canis*.

CONTRAINDICATIONS LOTRISONE Cream is contraindicated in patients who are sensitive to clotrimazole, betamethasone dipropionate, other corticosteroids or imidazoles, or to any ingredient in this preparation.

PRECAUTIONS **General** Systemic absorption of topical corticosteroids has produced reversible hypothalamic-pituitary-adrenal (HPA) axis suppression, manifestations of Cushing's syndrome, hyperglycemia, and glucosuria in some patients.

Conditions which augment systemic absorption include the application of the more potent steroids, use over large surface areas, prolonged use, and the addition of occlusive dressings. (See **DOSAGE AND ADMINISTRATION** section.)

Therefore, patients receiving a large dose of a potent topical steroid applied to a large surface area should be evaluated periodically for evidence of HPA axis suppression by using the urinary free cortisol and ACTH stimulation tests. If HPA axis suppression is noted, an attempt should be made to withdraw the drug, to reduce the frequency of application, or to substitute a less potent steroid.

Recovery of HPA axis function is generally prompt and complete upon discontinuation of the drug. Infrequently, signs and symptoms of steroid withdrawal may occur, requiring supplemental systemic corticosteroids.

Children may absorb proportionally larger amounts of topical corticosteroids and thus be more susceptible to systemic toxicity. (See **PRECAUTIONS-Pediatric Use.**)

If irritation or hypersensitivity develops with the use of LOTRISONE Cream, treatment should be discontinued and appropriate therapy instituted.

Information for Patients Patients using LOTRISONE Cream should receive the following information and instructions:

1. This medication is to be used as directed by the physician. It is for external use only. Avoid contact with the eyes.
2. The medication is to be used for the full prescribed treatment time, even though the symptoms may have improved. Notify the physician if there is no improvement after 1 week of treatment for tinea cruris or tinea corporis, or after 2 weeks for tinea pedis.
3. Patients should be advised not to use this medication for any disorder other than for which it was prescribed.
4. The treated skin areas should not be bandaged or otherwise covered or wrapped as to be occluded. (See **DOSAGE AND ADMINISTRATION** section.)
5. When using this medication in the groin area, patients should be advised to use the medication for 2 weeks only, and to apply the cream sparingly. The physician should be notified if the condition persists after 2 weeks. Patients should also be advised to wear loose fitting clothing. (See **DOSAGE AND ADMINISTRATION** section.)
6. Patients should report any signs of local adverse reactions.
7. Patients should avoid sources of infection or reinfection.

Laboratory Tests If there is a lack of response to LOTRISONE Cream, appropriate microbiological studies should be repeated to confirm the diagnosis and rule out other pathogens before instituting another course of antimycotic therapy.

The following tests may be helpful in evaluating HPA axis suppression due to the corticosteroid component:

Urinary free cortisol test

ACTH stimulation test

Carcinogenesis, Mutagenesis, Impairment of Fertility There are no animal or laboratory studies with the combination clotrimazole and betamethasone dipropionate to evaluate carcinogenesis, mutagenesis, or impairment of fertility.

An 18-month oral dosing study with clotrimazole in rats has not revealed any carcinogenic effect.

In tests for mutagenesis, chromosomes of the spermatophores of Chinese hamsters which had been exposed to clotrimazole were examined for structural changes during the metaphase. Prior to testing, the hamsters had received five oral clotrimazole doses of 100 mg/kg body weight. The results of this study showed that clotrimazole had no mutagenic effect.

Pregnancy Category C There have been no teratogenic studies performed with the combination clotrimazole and betamethasone dipropionate.

Studies in pregnant rats with intravaginal doses up to 100 mg/kg have revealed no evidence of harm to the fetus due to clotrimazole.

High oral doses of clotrimazole in rats and mice ranging from 50 to 120 mg/kg resulted in embryotoxicity (possibly secondary to maternal toxicity), impairment of mating, decreased litter size and number of viable young and decreased pup survival to weaning. However, clotrimazole was not teratogenic in mice, rabbits, and rats at oral doses up to 200, 180 and 100 mg/kg, respectively. Oral absorption in the rat amounts to approximately 90% of the administered dose.

Corticosteroids are generally teratogenic in laboratory animals when administered systemically at relatively low dosage levels. The more potent corticosteroids have been shown to be teratogenic after dermal application in laboratory animals.

There are no adequate and well-controlled studies in pregnant women on teratogenic effects from a topically applied combination of clotrimazole and betamethasone dipropionate. Therefore, LOTRISONE Cream should be used during pregnancy only if the potential benefit justifies the potential risk to the fetus.

Drugs containing corticosteroids should not be used extensively on pregnant patients, in large amounts, or for prolonged periods of time.

Nursing Mothers It is not known whether this drug is excreted in human milk. Because many drugs are excreted in human milk, caution should be exercised when LOTRISONE Cream is used by a nursing woman.

Pediatric Use Safety and effectiveness in children below the age of 12 have not been established with LOTRISONE Cream.

Pediatric patients may demonstrate greater susceptibility to topical corticosteroid-induced HPA axis suppression and Cushing's syndrome than mature patients because of a larger skin surface area to body weight ratio.

Hypothalamic-pituitary-adrenal (HPA) axis suppression, Cushing's syndrome, and intracranial hypertension have been reported in children receiving topical corticosteroids. Manifestations of adrenal suppression in children include linear growth retardation, delayed weight gain, low plasma cortisol levels, and absence of response to ACTH stimulation. Manifestations of intracranial hypertension include bulging fontanelles, headaches, and bilateral papilledema.

Administration of topical dermatologics containing a corticosteroid to children should be limited to the least amount compatible with an effective therapeutic regimen. Chronic corticosteroid therapy may interfere with the growth and development of children.

The use of LOTRISONE Cream in diaper dermatitis is not recommended.

ADVERSE REACTIONS The following adverse reactions have been reported in connection with the use of LOTRISONE Cream: paresthesia in 5 of 270 patients, maculopapular rash, edema, and secondary infection, each in 1 of 270 patients.

Adverse reactions reported with the use of clotrimazole are as follows: erythema, stinging, blistering, peeling, edema, pruritus, urticaria, and general irritation of the skin.

The following local adverse reactions are reported infrequently when topical corticosteroids are used as recommended. These reactions are listed in an approximate decreasing order of occurrence: burning, itching, irritation, dryness, folliculitis, hypertrichosis, acneiform eruptions, hypopigmentation, perioral dermatitis, allergic contact dermatitis, maceration of the skin, secondary infection, skin atrophy, striae, and miliaria.

OVERDOSAGE Acute overdosage with topical application of LOTRISONE Cream is unlikely and would not be expected to lead to a life-threatening situation.

Topically applied corticosteroids can be absorbed in sufficient amounts to produce systemic effects. (See **PRECAUTIONS.**)

DOSAGE AND ADMINISTRATION Gently massage sufficient LOTRISONE Cream into the affected and surrounding skin areas twice a day, in the morning and evening for 2 weeks in tinea cruris and tinea corporis, and for 4 weeks in tinea pedis. The use of LOTRISONE Cream for longer than 4 weeks is not recommended.

Clinical improvement, with relief of erythema and pruritus, usually occurs within 3 to 5 days of treatment. If a patient with tinea cruris and tinea corporis shows no clinical improvement after 1 week of treatment with LOTRISONE Cream, the diagnosis should be reviewed. In tinea pedis, the treatment should be applied for 2 weeks prior to making that decision.

Treatment with LOTRISONE Cream should be discontinued if the condition persists after 2 weeks in tinea cruris and tinea corporis, and after 4 weeks in tinea pedis. Alternate therapy may then be instituted with LOTRIMIN Cream, a product containing an antifungal only.

LOTRISONE Cream should <u>not</u> be used with occlusive dressings.

HOW SUPPLIED LOTRISONE Cream is supplied in 15-gram (NDC 0085-0924-01), and 45-gram tubes (NDC 0085-0924-02); boxes of one.
Store between 2° and 30°C (36° and 86°F).

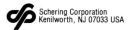 Schering Corporation
Kenilworth, NJ 07033 USA

Rev. 7/91   13182345

Copyright © 1984, 1991, Schering Corporation. All rights reserved.